Annihilate Allergies: Organic and Natural Methods for Safely Eliminate Allergies from Everyday Life

Disclaimer and Terms of Use: Effort has been made to ensure that the information in this book is accurate and complete, however, the author and the publisher do not warrant the accuracy of the information, text and graphics contained within the book due to the rapidly changing nature of science, research, known and unknown facts and internet. The Author and the publisher do not hold any responsibility for errors, omissions or contrary interpretation of the subject matter herein. This book is presented solely for motivational and informational purposes only.

Summary

Allergies are real and there are people who suffer from them worldwide. They may be seasonal or a bit permanent. Although over-the-counter drugs provide instant relief from these allergies, using natural healthy solutions has its advantages. You will not have any side effects that are common with the prescription drugs and you will be able to re-balance your immune system which may help in eliminating any allergic reaction in future. These are the reasons why many people are turning to healthy diets as a way of eliminating allergies.

We are going to help you in this journey by informing you of the different types of allergies people get, the foods that help to eliminating energy, the worst foods you should avoid when you have allergies, the steps to take in order to use healthy diet to successful do away with allergies and how to use the recommended foods to prepare healthy recipes that can help eliminate allergies.

Our aim is to show you what it means to go the healthy diet way in a bid to eliminate allergies and at the end of the day, it might help you in making an informed decision on whether you would be interested in trying it out or not. Enjoy reading!

Table of Contents

Introduction

Allergy is a common phenomenon. If you don't have it then someone close to you definitely does. It has gotten to a point where it is taken to be a normal thing yet that shouldn't be the case. No one wants to have a red runny nose, puffy eyes and all the other symptoms of allergies. When you have allergies then they influence your emotions and how you feel about yourself and you can't feel good about yourself when you feel terrible.

Many people resort to over the counter drugs to treat their allergies because they work fast. However, they forget that they have side effects especially when used over a long period of time. The use of natural means to eliminate allergies is fast gaining popularity among many people. This is because they are able to provide long term benefits to your immune system without causing it any harm.

If you have tried all means of eliminating allergies and failed then you might want to re-consider your diet. This is because out diet greatly contributes to a lot of reactions in our body. A healthy diet might just be what you need.

Chapter 1: Types of Allergies

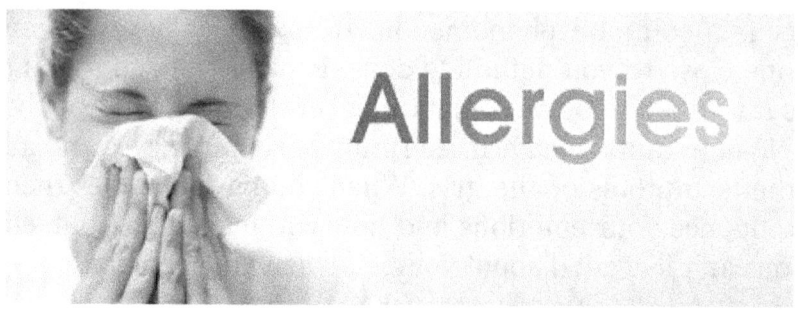

All allergies are a result of a hypersensitive reaction to a substance that is normally harmless. This doesn't mean that the different types of allergies are similar. For example, you might find that someone can go through an entire field of spring flowers without any negative effects but the mere thought of peanut can give him hives. It is therefore important to find out what causes your allergy in order to know how to prevent and treat it properly.

Allergies can be grouped according to their symptoms or according to the types of allergens that provoke those symptoms.

1. Anaphylaxis

This occurs when some specific allergens elicit a very dangerous response in the immune system. When your immune system experience sudden changes then this can affect various systems in your body such as the nervous system, your breathing mechanism and your cardiovascular system. Anaphylaxis can lower your blood pressure so much and make your tongue and throat to swell which hinders breathing. If a person experiencing anaphylaxis doesn't receive immediate medical attention to counter the reaction using epinephrine medicine then it can result in to death. Although this type of allergy is dangerous, the only consolation is that it is triggered by very few allergens and only a small number of people suffer from it.

The common allergens that trigger this reaction include insect stings, latex, eggs, injected anesthetics, shellfish, dye normally used in conducting radiology tests, tree nuts or peanuts and some antibiotics such as cephalosporin, penicillin and others that contain sulfa. In case you experience a hive or rash from any of these then avoid being exposed to them.

2. Allergic Rhinitis

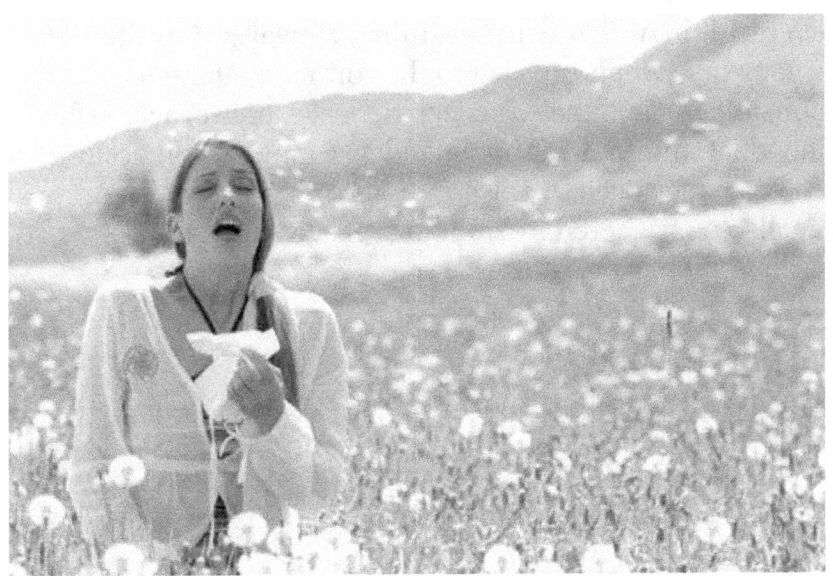

This refers to swelling, itching, inflammation and extreme secretions of the nose and sinuses. They are commonly referred to as "seasonal allergies" or "hay fever". This type of allergy is triggered when the triggers are inhaled for example pollens, cat or various animal dander, molds, dust containing proteins deposited by dust mites and proteins found on cockroaches or inside the remains of what they shed.

Airborne allergens are inhaled through the nose, eyes and throat and are responsible for production of large amounts of histamines responsible for itchiness, inflammation, sneezing, local swelling and the production of mucus taking place in the nose. Seasonal allergies occur during summer, spring or fall. You can find that someone can have an allergy allergic on one or all of these seasons. It goes down to the particular tree, plant or grass that you may be allergic to.

3. Asthma

Asthma is associated with inflammation and airtight airways which result in difficulty in breathing. However, the allergy may get worse when exposed to the common allergens responsible for this such as cockroaches, exercise, acid reflux, pollen, dust mites and animal dander. It might even occur when you experience strong emotions or high levels of stress. It can also be triggered by smoking tobacco and being exposed to various chemicals.

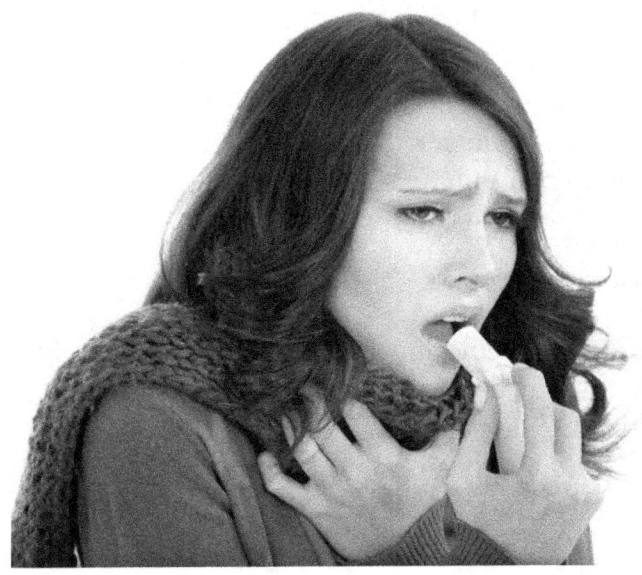

4. Skin allergies

Hives is a type of skin allergy and can be present in a variety of allergic reactions. Hives are rashes that are very itchy and can appear as small bumps or resemble the flat raised welt resembling a mosquito. If the allergic reaction gets worse then they expand. Hives are not common due to the fact they can be triggered by allergens in addition to exposure to heat and cold, excessive sweating or even physical pressure.

5. Eczema

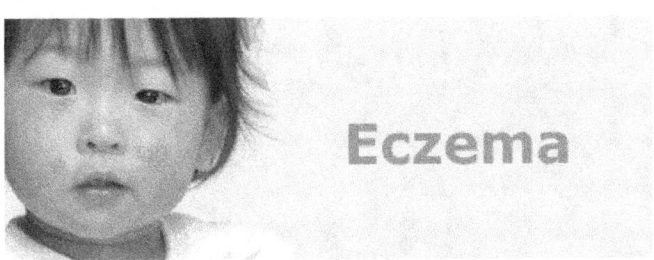

Eczema

Eczema is a condition whereby you develop an inflamed skin rash which comes with red skin, skin thickening and there are times when skin surface peels off in the dry areas. This is normally referred to as "scale". Sometimes eczema may appear as inflamed red patches that may release some seep clear fluid which may or may not be a result of allergy.

6. Contact Dermatitis

This is a rash that is red in color and is formed when your skin comes in contact with an allergen. Examples of the allergens responsible for this include poison sumac, cobalt, poison ivy, nickel, neomycin found in antibiotic skin ointment, poison oak and latex.

7. Food allergies

Food allergies affect a very small percentage of people which has been discovered to be 1% in adults, 2% in newborns and older children and 8% in preschool children. Food intolerances on the other hand are more frequent and lead to symptoms such as diarrhea, nausea and abdominal pain. Examples include being sensitive to caffeine or lactose. They are however not dangerous because they don't affect your immune system. Food allergies on the other hand can lead to anaphylaxis.

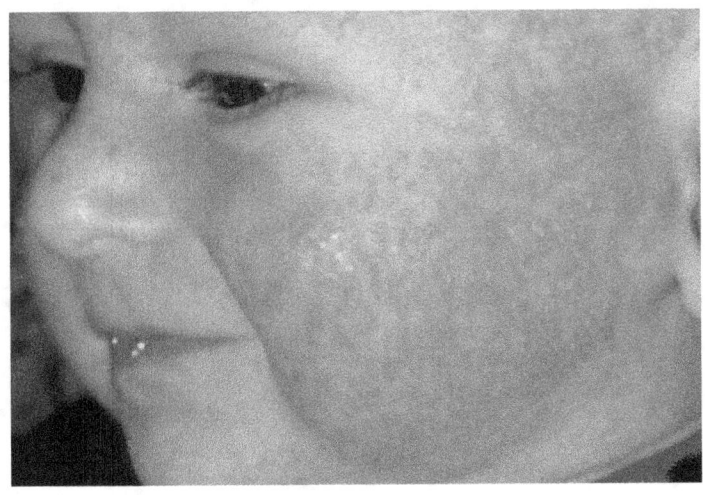

Children can outgrow food allergies such as allergy to cow's milk. However, there are some such as allergies to fish and peanuts that normally continue in to adulthood. If you have food allergy then you have to be cautious about what you eat.

8. Medical allergies

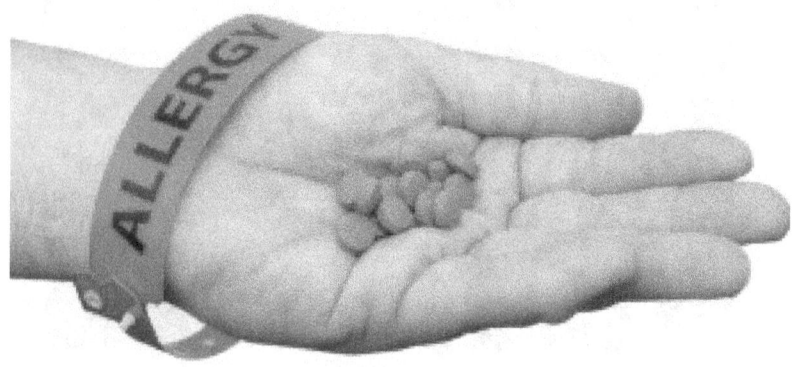

If you react to any medication then you should take it seriously even if it is not an allergic reaction. Health care providers take exceptional care when it comes to allergic reactions related to medications due to the fact that they can result in to anaphylaxis which is a type of reaction that is life threatening. There are some medications which are more likely to cause this reaction compared to others. Examples include cephalosporins and penicillin among others.

9. Insect venom allergies

When you have an insect bite, there is some venom that normally gets in your skin and this is what some people are allergic to. The most dangerous insect allergies are allergies to wasp stings, bee and hornet among others. There are reactions to some insects that are milder and an example includes a mosquito bite.

It is easy to notice a rash when you are bitten by an insect even if you are not allergic to insect venom. The rash may spread and may appear red or swell. You may experience hives and itching if you are allergic to insect bites. You need to seek medical attention in case you get this reaction before it develops in to anaphylaxis which is dangerous.

10.   Environmental allergies

This is allergy that is connected to dust mite, mold, animal dander, pollen, exposure to cockroach, allergic rhinitis, proteins and dust mite deposits. It means that they are influenced by your surroundings which you need to be aware of. The common types of reactions resulting from these allergens include asthma, allergic rhinitis and atopic dermatitis.

Chapter 2: Allergy Fighting Foods

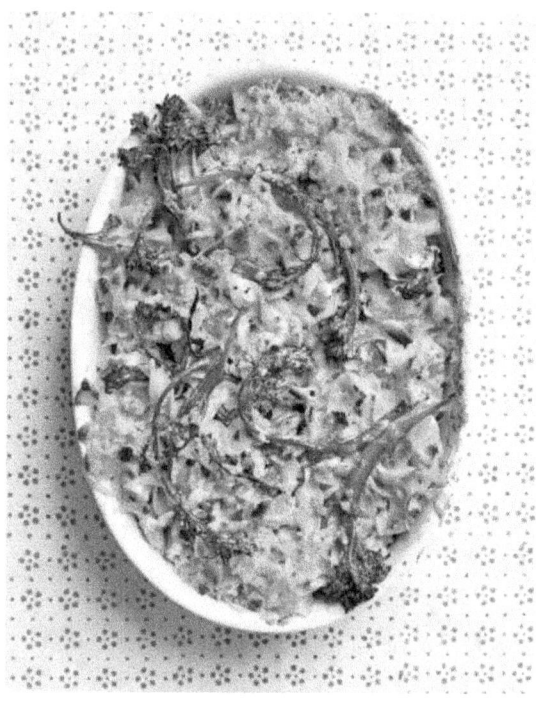

The best way to avoid the symptoms of your particular type of allergy is to avoiding triggering the allergy. However, when the allergy occurs then it is important to try and find ways of getting some relief from it. A good healthy diet has always been important in controlling any medical condition and allergies too. According to research, there are some foods with the ability to fight allergies and they do this by dilating air passages, keeping underlying inflammation under control and by giving various relief effects. Examples of those foods include:

Probiotics

Research has shown that probiotics have both anti- allergic and anti-inflammatory effects especially when taken by pregnant or breastfeeding women. A recent study conducted concluded that mothers who drank milk with a probiotic supplement when pregnant and afterwards greatly reduced the chances of their babies having eczema by almost half. Eczema is a condition associated with various forms of allergies. An Italian study concluded that children between the ages of two and five who had allergic rhinitis experienced less allergic episodes after drinking fermented milk made with probiotic *Lactobacillus casei* for one year compared to those children who were given placebo.

Sinus clearing spices

Spicy foods that help to clear sinus have been discovered to be important in getting rid of allergy symptoms. I know this is the last thing you would have thought of but it works. However, this should not be taken to mean that all spices should be used to eliminate allergies because that won't work and it might even make things worse. The spices referred to here have a little kick to them and examples include fennel, hot mustard, Anise and horseradish among others. They are able to relieve you of your allergy due to the fact that they are natural decongestants. They stimulate the mucosal cilia in order for it to clear the congestion and therefore offer you relief. You can prepare recipes that have these spices or add them to your food in case you begin to feel stuffy.

Fruits high in Vitamin C

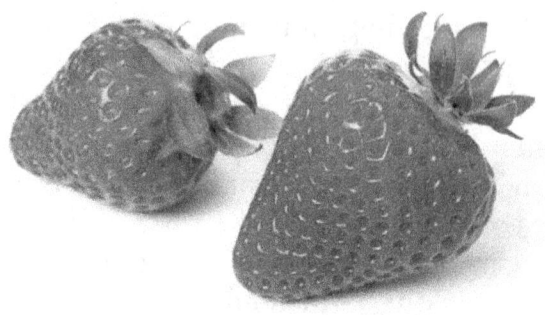

Histamine is what normally makes you experience hives, itchiness and various forms of discomforts when you are having an allergic reaction. When you take in Vitamin C, then it works by preventing the production of histamine by the inflammatory cells. According to studies, high amounts of vitamin C are important in both decreasing histamine and also in breaking it down much quickly and so you get energy when it is released. In addition to that, foods rich in vitamin C help to reduce inflammation too which works to underplay allergies and provide relief.

Vitamin C acts an oxidant which means that it is able to neutralize the inflammatory effects that free radicals give out. In simple terms food such as strawberries, watermelon, apples and oranges that contain high levels of vitamin C are good for reducing allergic response.

Bioflavonoids

Research has proven that bioflavonoids have the ability to relieve you of your allergy due to the fact that they are mast-cell stabilizers. They work by reducing the amount of cells that react to allergens. Mast cells are the ones that give out histamine. A bioflavonoid known as quercetin particularly stands out as being very strong with regards to fighting inflammation and offering relief from allergy. Tea, apples, red wine and onions are examples of the examples of good sources of quercetin.

Apples

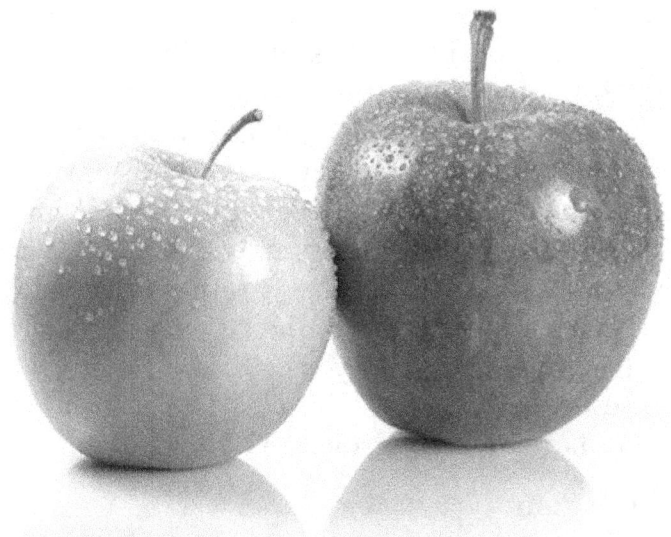

Eating an apple doesn't exactly get rid of pollen but research has found out that there are compounds inside an apple that can help to reduce the effect of the allergies. An apple a day can help to reduce your risk of getting asthma and allergies. There is an antioxidant known as quercetin that improves the functionality of your lungs and it exists on the skin of apples. It is also found in both onions and tomatoes.

Foods containing Magnesium

Wheat ban, almonds, kelp and cashews are examples of foods that are rich in magnesium that can give you allergy relief. Magnesium is important in relieving allergy due to the fact that it is an antihistamine and bronchodilator. It is therefore able to calm the bronchial tubes muscles and also the entire body. A study carried out by the Brigham Young University indicated that animals with a magnesium deficiency experience a greater amount of histamine in their system compared to animals that have the right amount of magnesium.

Food high in Vitamin E

There are various types of Vitamin E and the one particularly known as gamma-tocopherol has the ability to lower allergy-related inflammation. A study carried out by the Michigan State Unversity discovered that animals given high quantity of gamma-tocopherol and then allowed to breathe in deeply polluted air had nasal passages with a low amount of inflammation compared to the animals that weren't provided with the gamma tocopherol. What you have to know is that you have to take greater levels of the gamma tocopherol for it to be effective. For example, if you are taking soybean oil then you need several gallons of it in a day. You can choose to replace other fattier oils with soybean oil.

Cold-Water Fish

Cold water fish containing high levels of omega 3 fatty acids also contain anti-inflammatory effects. A good example of this fish is the salmon. Flaxseeds and walnuts are other sources of omega 3 fatty acids with inflammation fighting properties.

The only challenge with this is the fact that it requires a huge amount of omega 3 fatty acids to experience a small amount of benefit. You can make a commitment to eat fish more. Research shows that societies in which fish is readily available has showed that they have less allergic reactions.

Fresh fruits and vegetables

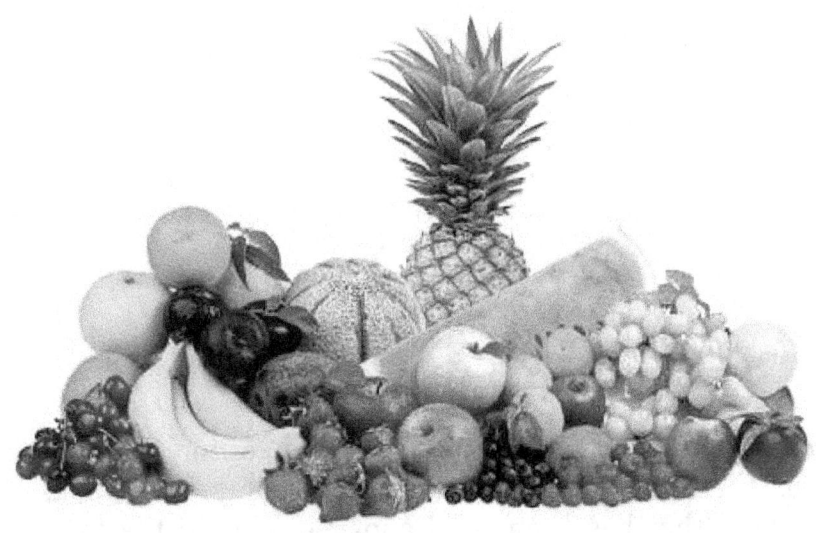

Fresh fruits and vegetables are the sure route to take if you want to better your diet and find relief from your allergy. It is possible due to the fact that they contain natural anti-inflammatory properties. Research was conducted on more than 400, 000 children and the results were that the children who ate plenty of tomatoes, ready vegetables and citrus fruits were at a lower risk of having shortness of breath and wheezing among other symptoms of rhinitis allergy. Another interesting finding was that the children who ate lots of bread and margarine were at a higher risk of getting wheeze.

Warm liquids

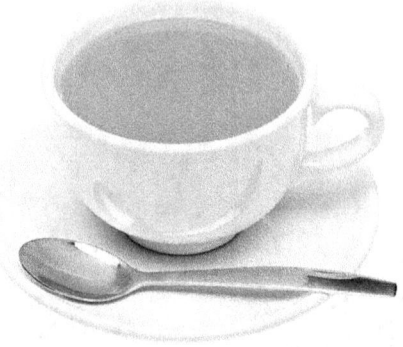

If your allergies appear in the form of congestion or coughing mucus then you should try taking a steamy drink. This is something that has been tried and it can be in the form of chicken soup or hot tea. This will help to reduce the mucus which will in turn ease congestion. In addition to that, it will keep you hydrated. If you don't feel like taking soup then you can even inhale a steam shower.

Red grapes

Red grapes contain an antioxidant known as resveratrol and it is where red wine derives its amazing name. This antioxidant contains anti-inflammatory powers important in reducing the symptoms of allergy symptoms. A study conducted on children in Crete concluded that taking fruits such as apples, grapes, tomatoes leads to a lower rate of wheezing and various symptoms of nasal allergy

Worst foods for allergies

After knowing the type of allergy you have then the next step is finding ways of avoiding triggering a reaction. The allergen responsible for your reaction is often mistaken by your immune system for being a threat and so the body responds by releasing histamine in a bid to protect you and this is what is responsible for the symptoms you experience.

Although you can try to avoid what triggers your reaction, this is a bit challenging when it comes to food allergy. Although staying away from the foods that triggers these reactions prevents you from getting a terrible reaction, it is not easy because you may not even know that are you consuming food with the particular allergen. This is especially if you are eating from a restaurant or are not the one who prepared the food.

By knowing some of the foods you should eat if you have allergies and the ones you should avoid, you can be able to control your allergic reaction.

Celery

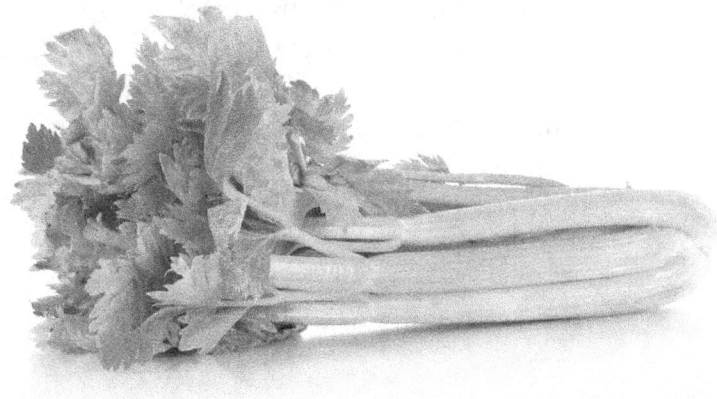

Studies have found out that some common allergy that affects people during spring do originate the same group of foods or families of plants in addition to particular fruits and vegetables. This syndrome is known as oral allergy syndrome. These allergies are quite different in the sense that instead of making you sneeze or sniff like the other allergies, you experience itchy mouth or throat.

Wheat, corn and rice all qualify to be called grass and if you have an allergic reaction to grass then you might be affected by a number of foods. Examples of the fruits and vegetables you should stay away if you are allergic to grass include tomatoes, celery, melons and peaches. If you have ragweed allergy then melons, bananas, zucchini and cucumbers should be out of your list of fruits and vegetables to eat.

Spicy foods

Although we have stated that sinus clearing spices can help to alleviate allergy symptoms, this is not the case with all spicy foods. Spicy foods are generally bad for you if you have an allergy. You can even realize this when you eat a spicy dish and feel the way it reacts all the way to your sinuses. Capsaicin is the compound responsible for making hot peppers spicy and it is also a great trigger of allergies and it might make your eyes to water and give you a running nose. In other cases, you might even end up sneezing. The reactions from spicy foods take place in a different route from real allergies. Although they may be mild, stay away from them completely in case you notice that they are getting more serious.

Alcohol

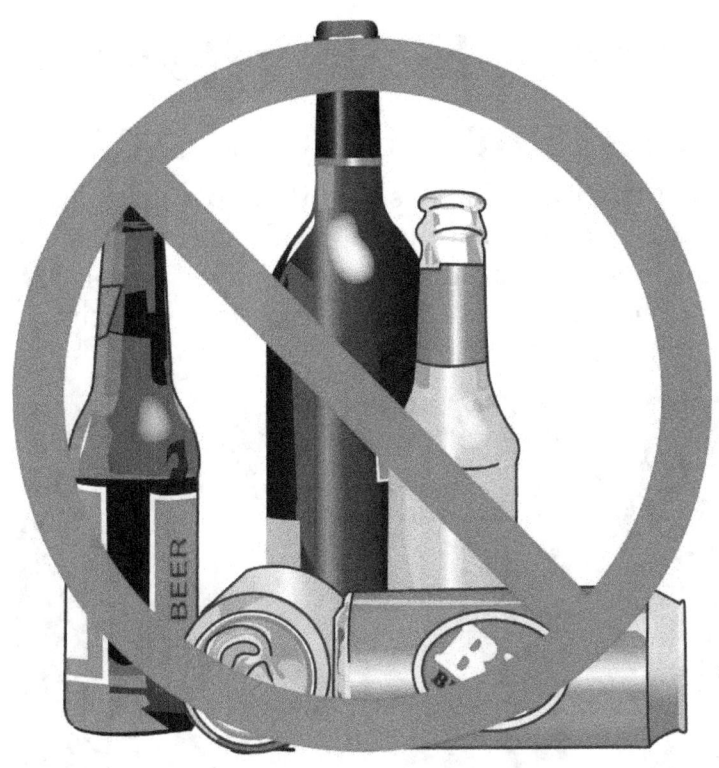

Have you ever noticed that you get a runny nose after taking a drink or more? This is due to the fact that alcohol has the ability to make blood vessels dilate and may worsen your allergy sniffles. The effect varies from one person to another and so you might slow down on the alcohol and monitor your reaction. In addition to that, alcohol contains histamine which naturally occurs during fermentation and we have seen about how dangerous histamine is on chapter one under "the types of allergies."

Chapter 3: Healthy Recipes for Eliminating Allergies Naturally

We have established that it is important to watch what you eat if you have an allergy in order to avoid triggering that allergy. You may be wondering about the recipes you can prepare when you have an allergy. You can try out these recipes.

Crockpot Lasagna

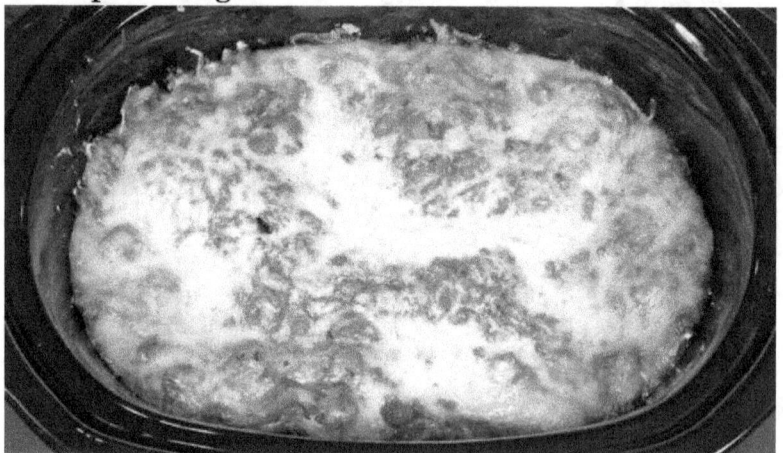

This is a main dish that you can make.

Ingredients

- 2 tablespoons of dried oregano
- ½ teaspoon of dried basil
- 3 cloves of pressed garlic
- 1 15 oz of firm tofu
- ¼ teaspoon of pepper
- ½ teaspoon of salt
- 2 cups of the Daiya mozzarella cheese. It should be shredded.

- 6 cups of fresh spinach, the young ones although they are optional.
- ¼ cup of parmesan, not grated.
- ¼ teaspoon of red pepper flakes. These are optional.
- 1 lb of cooked beef together with ½ onion. It should be ground. It is however optional.
- 1 pkg of lasagna noodles. Gluten free

Instructions

1. Mix together garlic, black pepper, tomatoes, basil, salt, oregano and red pepper inside a bowl.
2. Mix Daiya mozzarella cheese together with dairy free parmesan in a different bowl.
3. Spread a lean layer of sauce at the bottom of your cooker. Top it up with about 3 noodles.
4. Spread around one cup of sauce on your noodles and add some cooked meat and then spinach and ½ of the mixture of cheese. Keep repeating these layers until your crockpot become full. The noodles and sauce should be the final layers before sprinkling with mozzarella cheese.
5. Let the mixture cook for 3 ½ hours on low heat or until you are sure the lasagna has been thoroughly cooked.

This is a tasty mean but it is even tastier when it is reheated. Kids will love it when eaten with garlic bread. You can leave out the meat and spinach if you want. The number of layers are not quite important so you can do what you prefer. If it is not necessary to avoid taking wheat or gluten then you can use the regular lasagna noodle that is wheat based.

Avocado wrappers

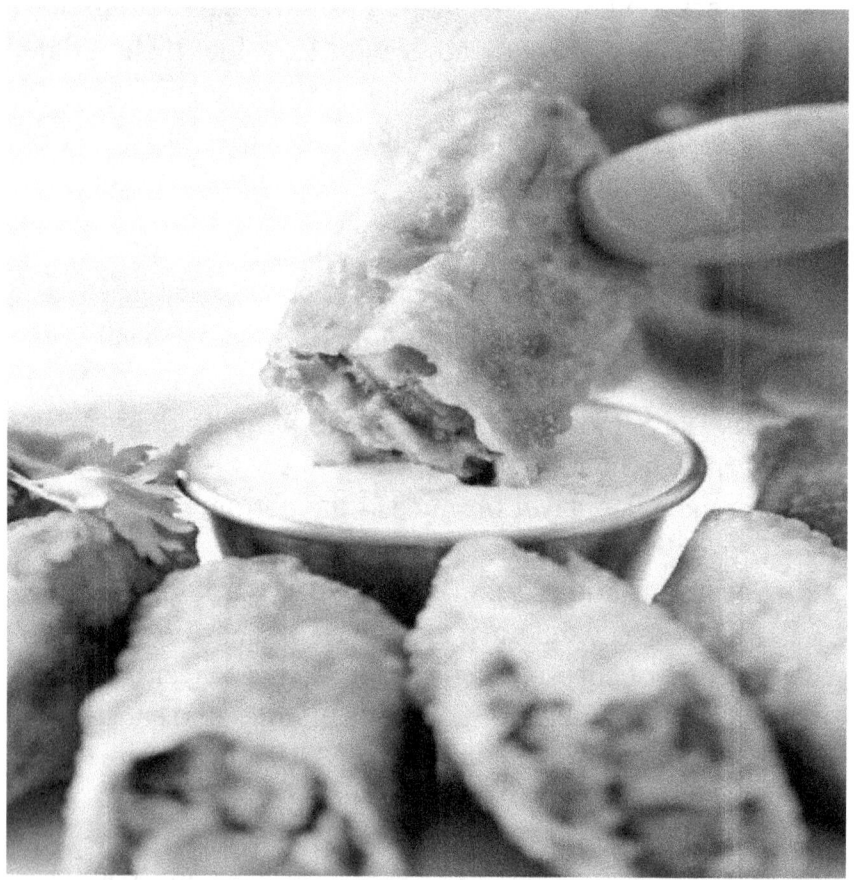

This is an appetizer that can serve twelve people.

Ingredients

- ¼ cup of sundried tomatoes which have been chopped and packed in oil.
- 1 scallion
- 1/8 teaspoon of black pepper
- 1 tablespoon of vegetable oil
- ¼ cup of cilantro, finely chopped and loosely packed

- 3 med of avocados that have been peeled, pitted and chopped in to ½
- 2 tablespoon of fresh lime juice
- ¼ tablespoon of salt
- 12 wonton oil wrappers used for deep frying

Instructions

1. Put one tablespoon of oil inside a saucepan and then sauté the scallion inside it and put on medium heat until they become soft and translucent. This can take about five minutes. Remove it and put aside in a cool place or under room temperature.
2. Mix cilantro, salt, avocado, lime juice and sun-dried tomatoes. Add the garlic and scallions and toss in order for them to combine.
3. Put an inch of vegetable oil and heat it on a temperature of 375° in a heavy skillet.
4. Put a tablespoon of the avocado mixture in the centre of a wrapper and do this for every wrapper. Dip your fingers inside some water and run it around your wrapper's edge in order to moisture it. Make the wrapper in a triangle by bringing together two opposite points. Pinch the edges using your fingers in order to crimp and seal all edges.
5. Deep fry them until they turn golden brown and you can do this by putting about two or three of them at once. Make sure you only turn them once. Give each side approximately a minute to cook. Use paper towels to drain.

You can then serve it immediately and include honey lime dipping sauce. You may substitute scallion for about ¼ of either purple or red onions and uncooked flour tortillas with egg free options. It is important to know that commercial wonton peppers normally have soy, egg and corn ingredients.

Vegan Zebra Cake

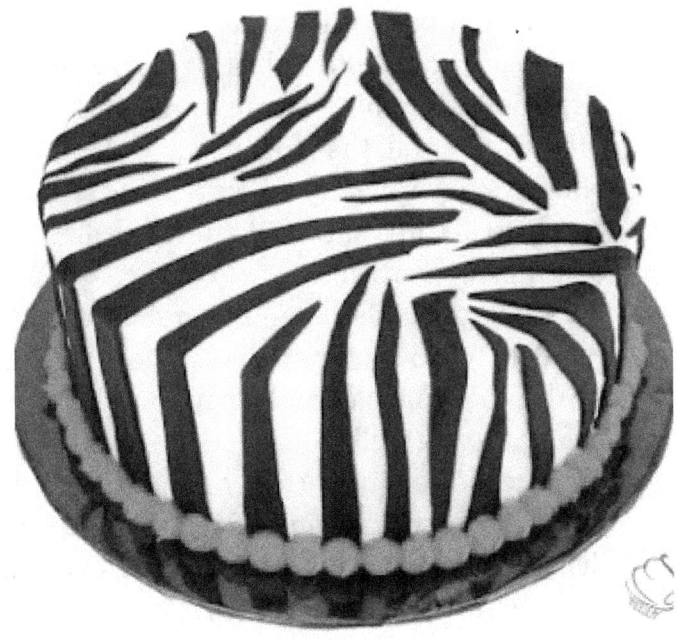

Ingredients

- 1 teaspoon of baking soda
- 1 ½ cups of flour
- 1 teaspoon of vanilla
- 1 cup of milk or its alternative
- 1 teaspoon of vanilla. This is optional
- 1 cup of sugar
- 1/3 cup of oil
- ½ teaspoons of salt
- 1 ½ to 1 tablespoons of cocoa powder

Instructions

1. Preheat the oven to a temperature of 350 °F. Prepare a cake pan of about 8" or 9". You can grease and flour your pan or use a cake release.
2. Mix together salt, flour, baking soda and sugar inside a large bowl. Combine the mixture by whisking.
3. Mix together oil, the milk alternative, vanilla and vinegar. Cover the dry works with wet ones and whisk it gently to attain a smooth batter. Be careful not to overmix or overbeat it.
4. Take half of the batter and pour it in another bowl. You can use the bowl that previously contained the wet works. Pick one half of the batter and ad cocoa to it before mixing well.
5. This step is very important because it should be able to give you the zebra stripes if you do it correctly. Take a disher preferably the 16 disher which is equivalent to an ice cream scoop and it can hold around 4oz. ¼ measure is okay. If you are using a measuring cup then ensure you scrap it every time after use to avoid mixing the banters.
6. Put the white batter first and place a disher of banter in the middle of the already prepared pan. Allow the batter to spread naturally and flow so you shouldn't move the pan.
7. Place a disher containing chocolate batter inside the white batter and do the same by letting it flow naturally too. Maintain an even rhythm when with the additions and don't let a long time pass in between. Continue doing this until you have used up all the batter.
8. Bake it at a temperature of 350 degrees for each one of them and you can do this for around 25-30 minutes for all them.

9. Remove the cake from the pan and leave it for some time on a rack in order to cool. Place it on a serving plate.

You can choose to frost it although it is very delicious the way it is. This moist cake is not too sweet or too chocolately so you shouldn't be afraid to try it if you are skeptical of sugary things. It goes well with coffee, tea or dessert. You can also take it as snack.

Although balsamic vinegar is used in this recipe, you can use any type of vinegar. The cake will come out a little darker due to the balsamic compared to when you are using light colored vinegar. You can leave out the vanilla in case you have added vanilla flavored milk alternative to it.

Sweet potato bread that is milk free, gluten free and egg free

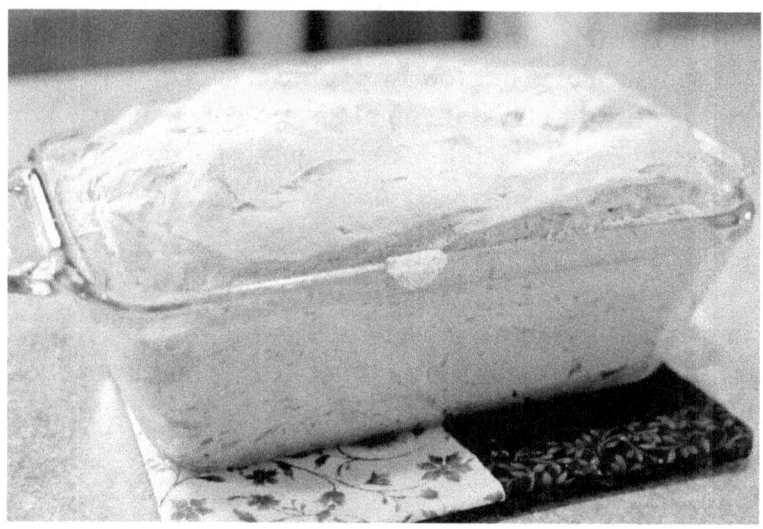

This is one loaf of bread.

Ingredients

- 1 box of mixed bread that is gluten free. This contains yeast packet
- ¼ cup of butter or oil
- 1 ¾ cups of milk alternative beverage, lukewarm
- ¾ cup of sweet potato puree

Instructions

1. Warm some milk on stove.
2. Mix sweet potato, milk, yeast and the oil or butter inside a standup mixer.
3. Add a cup of flour mixture at a time. Scratch the sides of every cup you add.
4. After adding all the flour, beat it for about two minutes under medium high speed.

5. Grease the loaf pan lightly and place the bread mixture on the pan.
6. Spread the bread mixture evenly inside the loaf pan using wet fingers.
7. Pre-heat the oven to about 350° F.
8. Keep aside the mixture in some warm place for like 20-40 minutes in order for it to rise or just leave it until it rises to the upper part of the loaf pan.
9. Bake for about 50-60 minutes.
10. Remove the bread from the loaf pan and put it on a cooling rack to cool.

Although grapeseed oil is used in this recipe, you can even use oil or butter. However, you should know that the recipe will no longer be milk free. Alternatively you can get soy-free margarines and milk free options. There are people who prefer the delicious coconut beverage as the milk alternative. If you don't like using eggs then you can go for sweet potato puree.

Spring vegetables and pancetta prepared with Quinoa Penne

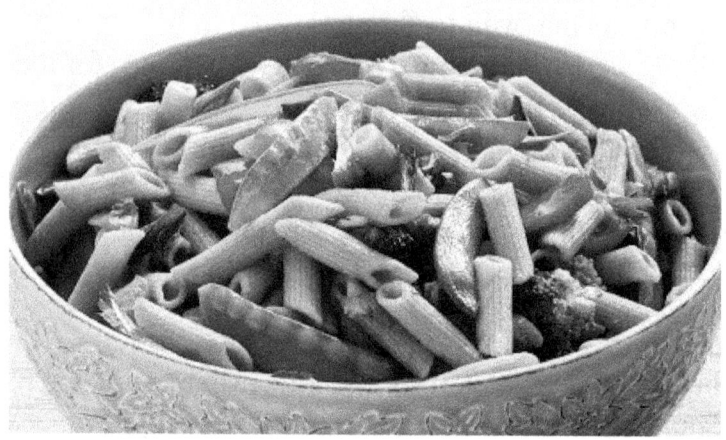

This meal serves four people and is gluten free and to allergens free

Ingredients

- 1 2 inch thick diced sliced of pancetta
- 1 small bunch of chopped basil
- 1 package of freshly cooked quinoa pasta
- ¼ cup of chopped chives
- 1 cup of snow peas, sugar snaps and broccoli florets
- Salt and pepper
- 1 piece each of diced yellow and red pepper

Instructions

1. Cook pancetta inside a big sauté pan until it turns golden brown. Remove it using slotted spoon and place it on a plate.

2. Blanch the snow peas, broccoli, blanch sugar snaps and salted water in a big pot containing salted water. Remove each ingredient in order to colander before draining.
3. Sauté the diced peppers inside dripping for about 4-5 minutes over medium heat. Add the blanched herbs, vegetables and cooked pasta and pancetta. Toss the mixture and warm it well before season it with salt and pepper. It is ready for serving.

If you are a vegetarian then you can leave out pancetta and also replace drippings with grapeseed oil (2 tablespoons).

Stuffed grape leaves prepared with Quinoa and Mint

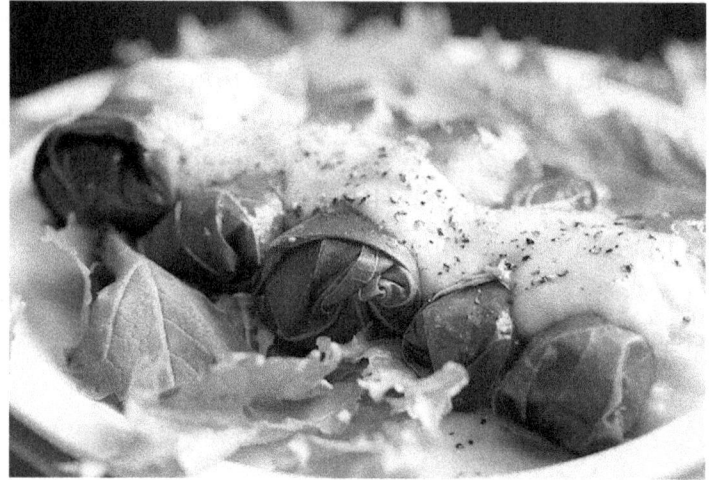

This recipe can serve between four to six people.

Ingredients

- 2 cups of allergen free vegetable stock (475 ml)
- 1 jar of drained grape leaves equivalent to about 30 leaves
- 2 cups of diced tomatoes equivalent to 475 ml
- 2 tablespoons of olive oil
- ½ cup of minced red onions equivalent to 125 ml
- 2 tablespoons of lemon juice
- 1 cup of raw quinoa equivalent to 250 ml
- 1 tablespoon of cumin
- Salt and pepper
- ½ cup of currants equivalent to 125 ml

Instructions

1. Cook quinoa in the vegetable stock in a medium saucepan. Cook it under medium heat until the quinoa is properly cooked and the liquid is absorbed.

2. Place the cooked quinoa in a big bowl and add the rest of the ingredients except for grape leaves. Stir properly and taste the seasoning.
3. Put the grape leaves on a flat place and put about 2 tablespoons of the filing on the center of every leaf.
4. Fold the length on one side and then on the other one too. Roll it in to a bundle starting from the bottom. Each should have the shape of a short fat cigar.
5. Continue doing this until you have used up all the filing. (Kids can love doing this)
6. Serve it with olives and hummus.

Lemon Chicken prepared with Asparagus salad and on Radicchio

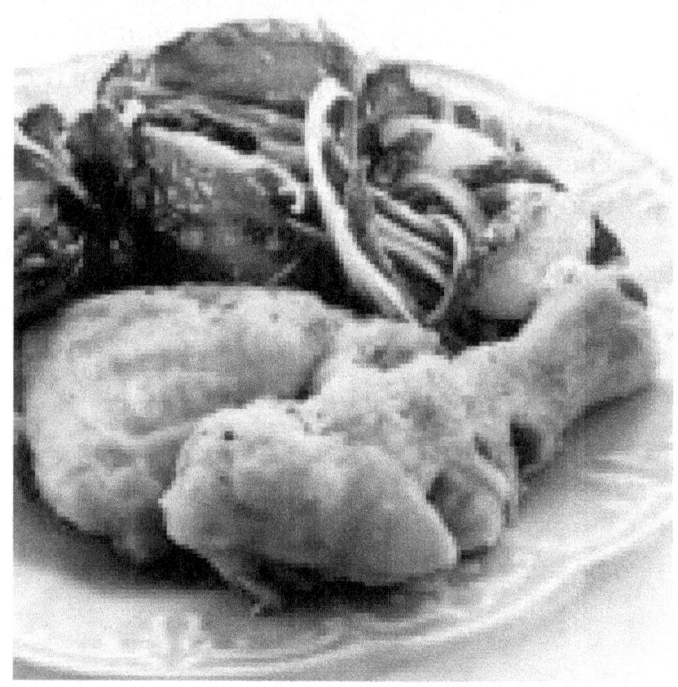

This meal can serve four people.

Ingredients

- 4 chicken thighs
- 2 bunches of trimmed asparagus
- 4 chicken legs
- 1 head of radicchio with separated leaves
- Zest of 2 lemons
- 1 small sliced red onion
- 2 tablespoons of olive oil
- 2 segmented oranges
- Salt and pepper

- 2tablespoons of rice wine vinegar, gluten free

Instructions

1. Heat the oven to a temperature of 400° F.
2. Use a sharp knife to score the chicken legs. Use olive oil, pepper, legs and thighs and salt using zest.
3. Let it roast in the oven for about 22-25 minutes until it is properly cooked.
4. Drizzle the asparagus with olive oil.
5. Roast it on the upper rack of the oven rack for about 8-10 minutes.
6. Serve the asparagus leaves and lemon chicken on the radicchio leaves.

Bistro split chicken prepared with baby potatoes over roasted fennel

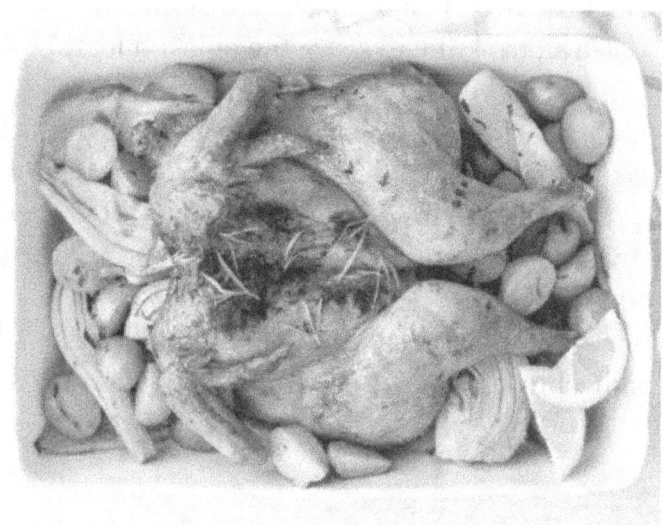

This French dish puts fragrant fennel, shallots, spring herbs and tiny potatoes to good use and serves four people. When you split a chicken then it allows for even roasting and a great presentation.

Ingredients

- 1 lb of young of halved, or fingerling potatoes equivalent to 450g
- 2 tablespoons of chopped fresh basil
- 2 medium of rinsed bulbs fennel each cut into 8 wedges with the ends removed
- ½ teaspoon of black pepper, freshly ground. Have some additional ones for chicken
- 3 peeled and quartered shallots
- 3 tablespoons of fresh and divided tarragon
- 4 tablespoons of divided oil
- 1 tablespoon of fresh chopped thyme

- 1.6-1.8 kg of chicken
- ½ cup of dry white wine equivalent to 120 ml
- Zest and juice of from 1 lemon

Instructions

1. Preheat the oven to temperatures of about 400° F and have the rack in the center while doing this.
2. Mix together the potatoes, ½ teaspoon of salt, fennel, 1 tablespoon of tarragon, shallots, ¼ teaspoon of pepper and 3 tablespoons of olive oil.
3. Rinse the chicken and pat it dry. Use kitchen shears or knife to divide the chicken down its backbone. Flip it and then press it down firmly using the palm of your hand. Do this on the breastbone in order to flatten it. Divide the chicken though do not separate the skin and the breast. Do this starting from the tail end.
4. Mix together 2 tablespoons of tarragon, thyme, lemon zest and basil inside a small bowl. Spread the zest herb mixture and massage it under the chicken skin using your fingers. Secure the chicken skin using toothpicks at the tail end if necessary.
5. Place the chicken cavity on the upper side of the rack over the vegetables. Use salt and pepper to season it generously. (¼ teaspoon of each is enough) mix wine and lemon and pour it over the chicken.
6. Roast the vegetables together with the chicken for about 15 minutes. Remove the chicken from the oven and flip it using tongs. Baste it with pan juices and then use 1 tablespoon of olive oil to brush it. Use about 1/8 teaspoons of salt and pepper for seasoning. Put it back in the oven and roast for another 15 minutes.
7. Lower the temperatures to about 325° F. Bake the vegetables and chicken under the reduced temperatures for about 1 hour until the skin becomes crispy, the

juices run clear and the temperatures on the thickest part of the chicken reaches 185° F. Don't disturb it during this time.

8. Remove the chicken and leave it for about 10 minutes and then carve it. Serve it together with the roasted vegetables and add the pan juices.

Thai- style rice rolls

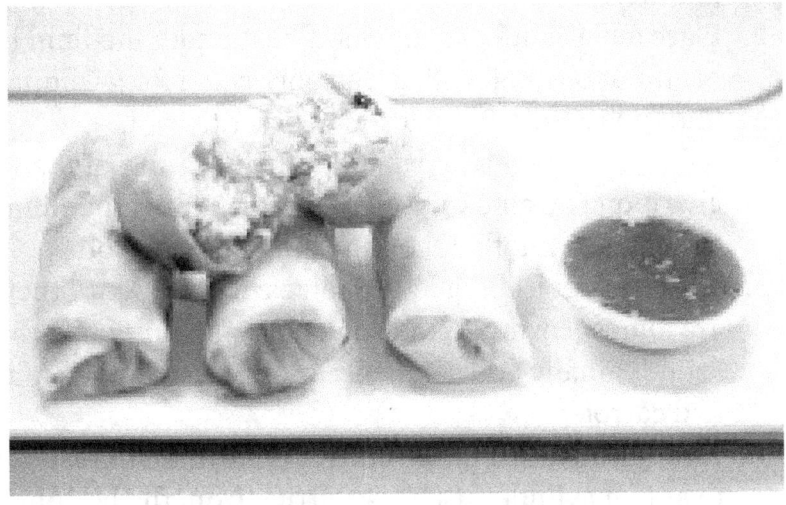

This recipe can accommodate 16-20 people.

Ingredients

- 1 lb of pork tenderloin equivalent to 450g and cut to form ¼ inch strips
- 1 tablespoon of minced, fresh ginger
- 1 iceberg lettuce
- 5 inch paper rounds of rice, 20 of them
- 1 tablespoon of Asian style chili sauce
- 1 apple which has been cut to form thin strips
- 2 tablespoons of olive oil
- 1 large carrot cut to form thin strips of three inches
- ½ cup of shredded mint leaves equivalent to 125 ml
- 1 tablespoon of minced garlic
- 1 seeded red pepper cut to form thin strips

Instructions

1. Mix together the garlic, chili sauce, pork and ginger in a bowl. Cover it and put it in the refrigerator for about 20 minutes.
2. Place a big sauté pan and let it heat under medium high heat. Put olive oil and let the pork sauté for 3-4 minutes until it is ready. Put it aside in order to cool.
3. Submerge every rice paper hound in warm water and give it one minute to become pliable. Place the rounds close to one another a clean damp piece of cloth.
4. Put layers of iceberg lettuce on each round until they are almost covered. Add some pork mixture on each round. Finally add some pieces of pepper, apple, mint and carrot.
5. Folds each round at the ends and roll it up to result in to a tight cylinder. Do this starting from the bottom end.
6. Halve the rounds and arrange them on a platter. Serve the meal using dipping sauce.

Sweet and sour

People have different tastes and depending on what you want, you can make this meal sweet and sour. There are some ingredients and steps you will have to include.

Ingredients

- ¼ of sulphite free brand of rice wine vinegar, seasoned.
- 6 finely chopped Thai basil leaves
- ¼ cup of olive oil
- 1 finely diced and deseeded red chili
- 1 teaspoon of sugar

Instructions

1. Mix together vinegar, oil and stir until all the sugar dissolves

2. Add the basil and chili

Final thoughts

Allergies are one of the things that might appear mild but are quite a bother and can even become life threatening. Have you ever thought of looking for a natural remedy for it? If you haven't because you didn't know they exist then now you do. You can make the choice to eliminate your allergies and do it in such a way that you achieve your goal and in a safe and healthy manner.

We have looked at the types of foods that can help you eliminate allergies naturally and you can use them to prepare your own recipes. We have gone ahead to provide you with some recipes you can try out too if you were at a loss concerning how to prepare the different types of foods important in eliminating allergies.

You no longer have to silently suffer with your allergies because there are healthy and natural treatments available. They say "prevention is better than cure". This is true and if you can avoid the allergens that trigger a reaction then it can be good. However, sometimes it is not easy to that especially if you don't have adequate and correct information to help you.

People are going the natural way and you can join too. If you find the information given in this book to be helpful then you can help a friend out who can also help another friend and with time, we'll find relief from our different types of allergies.

Yours sincerely,

Ruth Preston